The Brilliance of Bergamot Oil

Benefits, Properties, Applications, Studies & Recipes

by Ann Sullivan

Published in USA by:

Ann Sullivan
217 N. Seacrest Blvd #9
Boynton Beach
FL 33425

© Copyright 2015

ISBN-13: ISBN-13: 978-1544739359
ISBN-10: 1544739354

Table of Contents

Introduction

What are essential oils and how might they be used for therapeutic purposes?

Essential oils are ultra-potent oils extracted from plants and flowers that have been utilized in medicine for centuries. Presently, they are most commonly used to supplement pharmaceutical medication, but they can also be an effective alternative to pharmaceuticals in the event that you do not have access to them. Before dismissing essential oils, as a means to support the body's natural defenses against injuries and illness, take a look at the historical evidence of the oils' medicinal competence in practice. The average age-old medical text will demonstrate that essential oils, herbs, and plenty of other natural ingredients have, for thousands of years, successfully enhanced immune function to meet and defeat any number of ailments and injuries. Though traditional medicine is considered "alternative" now, it was once the gold standard. Perhaps it still should be, as these natural age-tested remedies can fortify the body's defenses against everything from simple maladies, like headaches, cuts, and bruises to serious diseases, like cancer.

Essential oils are deemed "essential," because the oils are composed of the "essence" of the plant. The difference between essential oils and other oils – like olive oil or vegetable oil, for instance – is that essential oils have high volatility and reduced fixation, which results in faster evaporation, enabling their popular use in aromatherapy. Even at high temperatures, olive and vegetable oils don't evaporate.

Essential oils are especially necessary when it comes to a major natural/man-made disaster or some potential viral outbreak. In these dire situations, we may not have quick access, or access at all, to our standard pharmaceutical supply; essential oils, along with other alternative medicines, will be our go-to health aids in the case of social collapse, viral outbreak, or devastating natural disaster. When medical access is null and void, alternatives to our modern-day standard are the only chance we have to keep pathogens at bay.

Most people do not realize that we already use essential oils every day. They are in perfumes, shampoos, soaps, ointments; they are even used in furniture polish. Why are they found in so many aromatic products? Well, essential oils are super concentrated aromatic liquids, so their aroma is remarkably strong. Putting this into perspective: to steam tea, use a few leaves of peppermint or juniper; to produce a single ounce of essential oil, five whole *pounds* of peppermint or juniper leaves are required. Some sources claim that to produce twelve pounds of essential oil would necessitate an acre of peppermint, juniper, or any other oil being produced en masse. Unlike vegetable oil, finding concentrated therapeutic-grade essential oils sold in bulk is uncommon; instead the oils are often sold in easily carried small, dark bottles, perfect for the GOOD bag (Get Out Of Dodge). That is precisely what this book is designed to accomplish – getting out of dodge with vital essential oils intact, in particular a good supply of Bergamot essential oil.

Why Bergamot, you ask? In order to get quickly up to speed on this most essential of oils, below we have provided a condensed synopsis of Bergamot, after which we will outline in greater detail the oil's history, properties, and common therapeutic uses, so that the consumer has a better understanding of the oil's benefits and applications. We have even provided supportive remedies for pure Bergamot, as well as blended recipes that incorporate the valuable oil. Chapter 3 will further detail past scientific research on Bergamot essential oil.

Now, let's get down to it – **Essential Oil 101: The Basics of Bergamot.**

Summary: Bergamot, or Citrus bergamia, has been used for thousands of years, with roots in oriental medicine. Historically, it was used to treat the digestive system and to help energy flow smoothly. During the Napoleonic age, Bergamot was often used in perfumes and colognes, a trend that still exists today.

Bergamot is not only valued for its pleasant scent; Bergamot essential oil has antiseptic and antibacterial properties that greatly benefit skin conditions.

Description: Bergamot oil is commonly extracted through steam distillation, or cold pressed. The citrus rind is often used. The oil is gold-green in color, thin in consistency, and has a medium fresh citrus scent.

Uses: Beyond those applications previously mentioned, additional uses for Bergamot essential oil include supporting the body's defenses against halitosis, itching, acne, boils, abscesses, cystitis, anxiety, cold sores, loss of appetite, psoriasis, indigestion, colic, oily skin, anorexia, inflammation, vaginal candida, and infections. When it comes to mood and emotion, Bergamot oil can help relieve stress, anxiety, fatigue, anger, depression, fear, loneliness and insecurity. It can stimulate confidence, happiness, and peace.

Properties: Anti-bacterial, antidepressant, anti-catarrhal, anti-tumorous, anti-inflammatory, antispasmodic, antiparasitic, antiseptic, anti-aging, immune-stimulant, sedative, analgesic, carminative, tonic, diuretic, digestive, vulnerary, and expectorant.

Application: Dilute 1:4 with a carrier oil. It can be applied topically, diffuse, or use as a dietary supplement.

Safety Precautions: Bergamot has been approved by the FDA for internal consumption, making it available for use as a dietary supplement. However, dilution is highly recommended if applying topically, as Bergamot can irritate sensitive skin. It is also phototoxic; avoid direct sunlight for up to 72 hours after application. Do not use on children under 5 years old.

Fun facts: Bergamot is so named, because it is said to have been brought by Columbus to Bergamo, a city in Northern Italy, from the Canary Islands. Bergamot has since been in regular use in Italian Medicine.

Chapter 1:
Benefits of Bergamot Essential Oil

Bergamot oil offers a number of therapeutic benefits; you may be wondering what these benefits are. In this chapter, we will take a closer look at the history of Bergamot and its many uses.

Cultivation of Bergamot

The Bergamot orange, or Citrus bergamia, is yellow like a lemon, but the size of an orange, and is probably a Citrus limetta/Citrus aurantium hybrid. The warm, humid temperatures of the Ionian Sea coastal regions in Reggio Di Calabria, Italy are perfect for the cultivation of this fruit, which is why these areas are the primary source of production, and the fruit is even the emblem of the city. Over 80% of the global production of the fruit comes out of southern Italy, while Turkey and France also cultivate Bergamot, using it in the making of marmalade and essential oil, respectively. Turkey also uses the Bergamot orange in its sweet treat, Turkish delight. The fruit is used in the making of many other food and drink items, particularly desserts.

Blossoming during winter, lemon-like fruit grows on the small Bergamot trees and has a distinct taste with a bitterness that resides somewhere between a grapefruit and a lemon. Bergamot trees are also a common "companion plant," as they are believed to keep pests from getting at the roots of neighboring plants.

A History of Bergamot

The word, "Bergamot," was derived from the Italian city, Bergamo. Sometimes confused with Citrus limetta and Citrus medica, the aroma of Citrus bergamia is quite pronounced and is utilized in the making of Earl Grey tea.

Calabrian indigenous medicine has been known to use Bergamot juice to help treat malaria, while the leaves of the fruit have long been used by Native Americans to treat digestive issues.

It takes 100 oranges to produce around three ounces of essential oil. The purity of some Bergamot oils on the market has been called into question, enforcing the Italian government to control, test, and certify purity. A Quality Control Body was established in Reggio di Calabria exclusively to verify the essential oil's quality.

The aromatic skin produces an essence which is utilized in tea and marmalade flavoring. The fruit is also routinely used as a flavor additive in the smokeless tobacco product called snus, which is popular in Norway and Sweden, and in dry nasal snuff. Reggio Calabria also uses the fruit to produce a digestive liqueur, called Liquore al Bergamotto. Oddly enough, the fruit itself, is not commonly eaten.

The peel of the fruit is also used in the making of perfumes and other fragrant products. The scent of Bergamot is highly complementary to other aromas commonly used in perfumes. In fact, Bergamot is used in around a third of colognes for men and around half of perfumes for women. The fruit's essence was prominent in the making of Eau de Cologne during the 18th century, which is also the first documented use of the oil as fragrance.

Chemical Components

In order to generate the essential oil from the Bergamot fruit, the rind must be cold pressed. This results in the oil's key chemical components, which are primarily linalyl acetate, limonene, linalool, β-pinene and γ-terpinene. Bergamot juice also includes melitidin, brutieridin, neoeriocitrin, neohesperidin, naringin, and ponceritin.

The polyphenols, melitidin, and brutieridin, exist in no other citrus fruits, and similarly to statins, they are known to suppress cholesterol biosynthesis. The Bergamottin, combined with 6',7'-dihydroxyBergamottin, is suspected of producing the metabolic effect of grapefruit juice when taken with pharmaceutical drugs. .

Main Properties of Bergamot Essential Oil

Along with the properties previously mentioned in the introduction, Bergamot oil possesses **anti-bacterial, anti-depressant, anti-catarrhal, anti-tumorous, anti-inflammatory, antispasmodic, antiparasitic, antiseptic, anti-aging, immune-stimulant, sedative, analgesic, carminative, tonic, diuretic, digestive, vulnerary, and expectorant** properties. With such a versatile range, Bergamot is well equipped to fight off any pathogen in the body.

Bergamot, as mentioned, is composed of linalyl acetate, limonene, linalool, β-pinene and γ-terpinene. These components are what instill the enormously beneficial properties within Bergamot essential oil. We will outline these properties below.

Antibacterial

Bergamot's antibacterial properties make it a powerful protectant against diseases produced by bacteria, such as oral, digestive, and urinary tract bacterial infection. What is great is that, unlike some prescription drugs, Bergamot has no ill effects on bodily health, or on the healthy natural flora that exists within the stomach and intestines. A study analyzing Bergamot's antibacterial properties can be read here.

Antidepressant

When it comes to psychological issues, the uplifting scent of Bergamot combats negative thoughts, thereby supporting relief from depression. A study on Bergamot's anti-anxiety properties can be found here and its effects on stress, here.

Anti-catarrhal

Catarrhal inflammation occurs when the mucus membranes in the body's airways, or cavity, are inflamed. This can cause a lot of mucus and white blood cells as the result of an infection. The symptom comes with coughs, the common cold, infections of the ear, adenoids, tonsils, and sinus. The phlegm issue can potentially become chronic; addressing it early on with an anti-catarrhal, like Bergamot, is a proactive measure to take towards recovery.

Anti-inflammatory

External or internal inflammation can be reduced through the use of Bergamot essential oil. For instance, if a patient has swollen fingers from arthritis, or a swollen knee from a sport's injury, oral application of Bergamot essential oil may decrease irritation, while also soothing the pain that accompanies inflammation.

Antispasmodic

The antispasmodic properties of Bergamot oil make it beneficial to such health issues as chronic coughing, and other respiratory conditions, along with surgical processes, such as colonoscopy and gastroscopy.

Antiparasitic

Parasites include such mites as fleas, bedbugs, tapeworms, mosquitoes, and lice – pretty much any irritating insect, internal or external, which feeds off the body in one way or another. The human body is a tasty meal to parasites, which can sometimes lead to the transmission of communicable diseases through their feasting off various meals. Bergamot is the answer. Its antiparasitic properties will support the body in combating mosquitoes, fleas, bedbugs, and lice when applied topically, and intestinal worms when taken orally, which is why Bergamot is commonly used in insect repellents.

Antiseptic

The antiseptic and disinfectant properties of Bergamot essential oil can be reaped topically, applied directly to wounds, or even through burning; the smoke from the oil may help destroy airborne germs. Internal use will help keep the wounds from becoming infections, while external use will inhibit tetanus.

Anti-aging

No need for those spliced-together anti-aging pills;

Bergamot essential oil has been shown to help decelerate the process of aging, by supporting the body's natural function when fighting the deterioration of cells with the oil's high number of antioxidants.

Immune System Booster

Bergamot is a superb immune system support which boosts circulation and increases white blood cell count. The oil's chemical trio of menthol, camphor, and carvacrol deliver Bergamot's incredible antifungal, antibacterial, and antiviral properties, making it akin to an immune shield braced to fight off angry bacterial strains, like salmonella, E. coli, and staph infections. With such strong armor, this immune stimulant will ensure that your body is better prepared to protect against deadly viral infections.

Sedative

As a sedative, Bergamot sedates and calms by reducing anxiety, excitement, or irritability. Though sedatives alone do not alleviate pain, they do calm the patient, making them less stressed and more compliant.

Analgesic

Bergamot's analgesic qualities make it an effective supplement for pain relief to be used in supporting relief from headache, sprains, injuries, wounds, scars, bruises, burns, and arthritis. It is a surefire aid to any sports muscle sprain, or recovery pain from surgery. A study on Bergamot's effect on pain relief can be found here.

Carminative

By supporting the reduction of excess gas buildup and/or removal of gas from the intestines, Bergamot essential oil provides relief from abdominal pain, excess sweating, and uncomfortable indigestion.

Tonic

Bergamot essential oil benefits each of the body's systems, whether nervous, digestive, respiratory, or excretory; making it an unbeatable general tonic. The oil also supports the immune system by helping the body absorb nutrients.

Diuretic

For those looking to lose water weight and reduce blood pressure, Bergamot essential oil is your weight loss enhancing agent. The oil stimulates urination, promoting not only the loss of water weight, but the loss of fats, uric acid, sodium, and other body toxins.

Digestive

By boosting the production of absorptive enzymes, the digestibility of nutrients, and the secretion of digestive juices, Bergamot essential oil aids the digestive tract significantly, which can have a great impact on the body's overall health by increasing those nutrients absorbed from food.

Vulnerary

Whether you want to support the body's defenses against

ulcers, cuts, or any internal or external wound, Bergamot essential oil can be diluted with a skin cream, and applied to expedite the process of healing while also protecting the wound from becoming infected.

Expectorant

Throat or respiratory infections can be relieved through the use of Bergamot essential oil. Acting as an expectorant, Bergamot helps break up and destroy the phlegm and mucus buildup that accompanies sinuses or respiratory infections. Inflamed throat and lungs, as well as coughing, can also be relieved through the use of this oil.

Common Medicinal Uses

With thousands of years of history rooted in oriental medicine, Bergamot was used to support the digestive system and to help energy flow smoothly. In particular, the scent of Bergamot was valued across ages. During the Napoleonic period, perfumes and colognes prominently featured Bergamot, a continuing trend in the modern day. The oil's properties also promote healthy skin. Below are a few more ways in which Bergamot can play a role in your body's overall health.

Stress Disorders

Whether it be physical stress or mental stress, Bergamot's fresh aroma, alongside its therapeutic properties, enable its use in the support of stress disorders; upset nerves, anxiety, melancholy, and depression. It can help soothe mental fatigue and the chronic fatigue that comes with it. The oil is said to stimulate clarity and strengthen overall mental well-being.

Insect Repellant

It is not necessary to be covered in a sticky bug spray to keep the mosquitoes at bay; Bergamot oil is a match for even the peskiest of bugs. Whether diffused in the buggy infested area, or applied topically with a few drops in a favorite skin cream, the strong insecticidal properties will stave off the bugs and smell great doing it. It is also used to keep bugs and other pests from eating at crops. This is why Bergamot is often seen in gardens as a "companion plant."

Perfume

The scent is used prominently as a perfume. Though insects do not seem to care for it, Bergamot has long been an active ingredient in perfumes and remains one to this day, appearing in half of women's perfumes (perhaps because the scent is a known aphrodisiac).

Bacterial Infections

For those of us who are susceptible to seasonal cold and flu viruses, providing our immune systems with a reliable mechanism of defense can mean the difference between illness and health. According to a study published in the *Journal of Applied Microbiology*, Bergamot essential oil does just that – it protects our immune system against bacterial infection, providing strong support when we need it most. Bergamot does this by combating bacterial strains, like

Enterococcus faecalis and Enterococcus faecium, both of which are resistant to the antibiotic, vancomycin, which usually treats bacterial infection. These bacteria can cause everything from meningitis to urinary tract infection to endocarditis. Bergamot oil in a sitz bath will support the body's natural defenses against these infections.

Maintaining Cholesterol Levels

According to the *Journal of Natural Products*, the polyphenols, melitidin and brutieridin, exist in no other citrus fruits, and similarly to statins, they are known to suppress cholesterol biosynthesis. This means that Bergamot may support the body's natural function in reducing cholesterol, something that affects 25% of Americans, aged 46 and older. Good cholesterol levels typically mean reduced risk of heart attack or stroke.

Skin Issues

With its antibacterial and antifungal properties, Bergamot essential oil promotes healthy, glowing skin by enhancing the body's natural healing process. When it comes to mouth ulcers, cold sores, herpes, chickenpox, shingles, and a litany of other skin issues, the oil combats bacterial growth while promoting sebum secretion balance within the body. The oil's disinfectant properties also allow for a clean healing process for skin conditions/wounds, reducing the amount of scarring. In fact, the *Journal of Antimicrobial Chemotherapy* published a study which tested Bergamot essential oil's effectiveness in inhibiting growth of various candida fungus strains with positive results.

Digestive Aid

A healthy digestive tract means a healthy body, so maintaining good digestion can have a significant impact on how we feel. Our digestive tract is between 25 - 30 feet long. If it is not working properly, then there is a chance that food can get caught up and begin to rot within the body. Bergamot effectively supports the digestive tracts natural function by helping induce bile flow throughout the digestive organs, which will benefit overall health.

Safety Precautions & Common Applications

Safety

Some adverse effects may evolve when using pure essential oils. Some essential oils should not be used when pregnant. Allergic reactions may occur, especially when applied topically. Always administer an allergy test before committing fully to topical application. When used with other medications, essential oils may react negatively. If a patient is on any current prescription medications, or has a chronic illness, such as high blood pressure, epilepsy, or liver disease, then researching the effects of essential oils against their personal medical history will eliminate any potential issues.

Blends

Oftentimes, essential oils are manufactured as blends of several pure oils. For instance, the Protective Essential Oil

Blend is a mix of cinnamon, clove, rosemary, and eucalyptus. This blend can be used to boost the immune system to help support the body's defenses against colds, viruses, and flus. The downside to blends is that the more oils added to the mix, the higher the probability the patient may react negatively to the blend if he/she is prone to allergies. There is also the possibility of phototoxicity when working with blends.

Regardless of these possible effects, essential oils are a viable option for supporting the body's defenses against a number of conditions. Those looking to enhance the maintenance of their own personal health, or that of their families, should become educated on the uses of essential oils, their natural remedies, and the methods of application. Only then can they begin building their kit of essential oils for survival.

Chapter 2:
Recipes for Bergamot Essential Oil

In this chapter, we will offer various recipes for Bergamot essential oil, both for pure Bergamot applications, and for blends. For pure supportive remedies, we have provided the appropriate application and dosage to help the body's natural function address specific ailments, from acne to worms. When it comes to blends, herbalists and aromatherapists often combine Bergamot essential oil with mandarin, clary sage, jasmine, frankincense, black pepper, geranium, cypress, vetiver, orange, ylang-ylang, sandalwood, and rosemary. It is a particularly complimentary oil, and blends well with just about anything, which is why it is so popular with the perfume industry. We will offer some fantastic supportive blending options in the second half of this chapter.

Pure Supportive Remedies

Acne

Enhance the body's natural ability to clear acne by diluting 2 drops of Bergamot essential oil in 4-5 drops of fractionated coconut oil and applying the combo to the affected area twice daily. Suggested application is before and after showering.

Addiction

To help combat addiction, dilute Bergamot essential oil in a 1:1 ratio with a carrier oil and apply topically, massaging over the solar plexus and the heart. You can also administer aromatically, diffusing throughout the home, or inhaling directly from the bottle.

Agitation

Agitation can be calmed by directly inhaling Bergamot essential oil. Pour a drop into the hands, rub palms together, cup them over nose and breathe.

Boils

Help eliminate boils by diluting Bergamot essential oil in a 1:4 ratio with a carrier oil and applying topically over the affected area.

Brain Injury

Support the body's natural defenses against brain injury by diffusing Bergamot essential oil throughout the room. Place

a drop on the patient's shirt collar, or pillow. Dilute
Bergamot essential oil in a 1:4 ratio with a carrier oil and
massage into scalp, neck, and shoulders.

Cold Sores

Strengthen the body's defenses against cold sores by
diluting Bergamot essential oil in a 1:4 ratio with a carrier
oil; dab directly onto the cold sore, or apply as a lip balm, if
you feel a cold sore coming on.

Colic

Colic can be alleviated through topical application. Dilute
Bergamot essential oil in a 1:4 ratio with a carrier oil and
massage into the soles of the feet twice daily.

Compulsions

Apply one drop to the feet, and one drop over the solar
plexus, 1-2 times a day in conjunction with inner work.

Confidence

To help boost confidence dilute Bergamot essential oil in a
1:4 ratio with a carrier oil and apply topically, massaging
over the abdomen several times daily. Administer
aromatically, diffusing throughout the home, or inhaling
directly from the bottle.

Depression

Support the body's natural defenses against depression by
steaming two drops of Bergamot essential oil in a pan of

water. Remove the steaming pan from the stove, pour into a bowl, place a towel over the head and inhale. If initially unsuccessful, reheat water and use again without adding more oil. Dilute Bergamot in a 1:4 ratio with a carrier oil and apply topically, massaging into the abdomen several times daily.

Digestion

To aid digestion place a drop in drinking water, or incorporate into cooking. Apply topically by diluting Bergamot essential oil in a 1:4 ratio with a carrier oil and massaging it into the abdomen before each meal.

Eczema

Help clear up eczema by diluting Bergamot essential oil in a 1:4 ratio with a carrier oil and applying topically to the affected area.

Empowerment

Get empowered by diluting Bergamot essential oil in a 1:1 ratio with a carrier oil and applying topically, massaging over the abdomen several times daily. Administer aromatically; pour a drop into hands, rub palms together, cup them over nose and breathe.

Exhaustion

To help ease physical or mental exhaustion dilute Bergamot essential oil in a 1:4 ratio with a carrier oil and apply topically, massaging the oil into the reflex points of the feet.

Administer aromatically, diffusing Bergamot throughout the home, or inhaling directly from the bottle. Additionally, throughout the day, add a drop to drinking water.

Fears

Stamp out those fears by diluting Bergamot essential oil in a 1:4 ratio with a carrier oil and applying topically, massaging over the abdomen several times daily. Administer aromatically; pour a drop into hands, rub palms together, cup them over nose and breathe.

Grief/Sadness

To relieve grief or sadness directly inhale Bergamot essential oil from the bottle. Pour a drop into hands, rub palms together, cup them over nose and breathe for a minute or more.

Indigestion

Bergamot aids the digestive tract and can be taken orally or topically. Place a drop into drinking water for internal administration, or by diluting the oil in a 1:1 ratio with a carrier oil, and applying topically to the abdomen in a clockwise motion before each meal. Diffuse throughout the home.

Infection

To enhance the body's ability to fight off infections dilute Bergamot essential oil in a 1:4 with a carrier oil and apply topically to the affected area, or to the soles of the feet.

Diffuse throughout the room, whichever application is more appropriate to the specific infection, internal or external.

Intestinal Parasites

Help the body rid itself of intestinal parasites by diluting Bergamot essential oil in a 1:4 ratio with a carrier oil and massaging it into the abdomen and the soles of the feet. Add a drop to drinking water.

Loss of Appetite

If grief, stress, illness, or depression causes appetite loss, then diffuse Bergamot essential oil throughout the home. Dilute Bergamot essential oil in a 1:4 ratio with a carrier oil and apply topically, massaging into the stomach before each meal.

Mental Stress

Support mental well-being by diluting Bergamot essential oil in a 1:4 ratio with a carrier oil and applying topically, massaging over the abdomen several times daily. Administer aromatically, diffusing Bergamot throughout the home, or inhaling directly from the bottle.

Oily Skin

Promote clear skin by diluting 1-2 drops of Bergamot essential oil in a 1:4 ratio with fractionated coconut oil and apply to a clean face. Diminish the appearance of blemishes by applying a drop to the affected area.

Physical Stress

If feeling physically stressed, then dilute Bergamot essential oil in a 1:4 ratio with a carrier oil and apply topically, massaging the oil into the reflex points of the feet. Administer aromatically, diffusing Bergamot throughout the home, or inhaling directly from the bottle. Additionally, throughout the day, add a drop to drinking water.

PMS

Help relieve menstrual cramps, or PMS related issues, by diluting Bergamot essential oil in a 1:4 ratio with a carrier oil and topically, massaging the oil into the lower abdomen, back, and into the reflex points of the feet. Support emotional balance by administering the oil aromatically, diffusing Bergamot throughout the home, or inhaling directly from the bottle.

Psoriasis

Bergamot can be used to support the body's natural defenses against all sorts of skin conditions, including psoriasis. Dilute Bergamot essential oil in a 1:4 ratio with a carrier oil and apply directly to the affected area twice daily.

Rheumatoid Arthritis

To combat the pain and inflammation of arthritis, dilute Bergamot essential oil in a 1:4 ratio with a carrier oil and apply topically, massaging the oil into the joints.

Scabies

Combat mites that cause scabies, help rid of the rash, and support the body's natural defenses in fighting infection by diluting Bergamot essential oil in a 1:4 ratio with a carrier oil and applying topically to the affected area several times daily

Sedative

Diffuse Bergamot essential oil throughout the home, or dilute Bergamot essential oil in a 1:4 ratio with a carrier oil, and apply topically in a full-body massage to take advantage of the oil's sedative properties.

Stress

To relieve stress directly inhale Bergamot essential oil from the bottle. Pour a drop into hands, rub palms together, cup them over nose and breathe for a minute or more. Apply topically by diluting Bergamot essential oil in a 1:4 ratio with a carrier oil and applying to the hands, feet, and abdomen.

Urinary Tract Infections

Support the body's natural defenses to eliminate urinary tract infections by diluting Bergamot essential oil in a 1:4 ratio with a carrier oil and massaging it into the soles of the feet, and over the kidneys, urethra, and bladder. Place 3-4 drops in a sitz bath and soak in it for 10-15 minutes, or add a couple drops to drinking water.

Varicose Veins

Reduce the appearance of varicose veins by diluting Bergamot essential oil in a 1:1 ratio with a carrier oil and applying topically in an upwards stroke towards the heart.

Worms

Support the body's natural defenses against worms by diluting Bergamot essential oil with a carrier oil and applying topically to the reflex points in the feet and over the abdomen.

Blends

Bacteria Killer

Ingredients

4 drops Lemon Essential Oil

4 drops Bergamot Essential Oil

2 drops Tea Tree Essential Oil

Directions

Diffuse blend throughout home to help destroy bacteria.

Calming Mood Mist

Ingredients

1 drop Frankincense Essential Oil

2 drops Bergamot Essential Oil

3 drops Lavender Essential Oil

4 ounces Distilled Water

Directions

Combine all ingredients in a small spray bottle. Tighten the lid and shake well. Spray into the air whenever in need of calm and relaxation. Shake well before each use.

Cleansing Facial Mask

Ingredients

1 drop Bergamot Essential Oil

2-3 drops Carrier Oil

2 tsps. Pink Clay

Rose Water (or Distilled Water)

Directions

For a cleansing face mask, wash face with warm water. Combine all ingredients in a small jar or bowl. Add only enough rose, or distilled, water to wet the clay. Apply the face mask evenly across face. Avoid the eyes. Let sit for 15-20 minutes then wash off with warm water. For best results, apply face mask twice weekly.

De-Stress Bath

Ingredients

4 drops Geranium Essential Oil

4 drops Bergamot Essential Oil

2 drops Vetiver Essential Oil

1 Tbsp. Grapeseed Oil (optional)

Directions

To wind down, de-stress, and combat anxiety, add all ingredients to bathwater and stir to disperse. Inhale deeply while soaking for 20 minutes, but avoid getting water in the eyes.

Moisturizing Scrub

Ingredients

¼ ounce Lavender Essential Oil

10 drops Bergamot Essential Oil

3 ounces Sea Salt

1-ounce Jojoba Oil

Directions

To create a moisturizing sea salt scrub, combine all ingredients in a small container, mixing until well blended. Set aside, letting the mixture sit covered overnight. Shake well then use as needed. Keep covered and shake well before each use.

Seasonal Depression Mood Booster

Ingredients

2 drops Ylang Ylang Essential Oil

4 drops Bergamot Essential Oil

4 drops Lemon Essential Oil

1 Tbsp. Grapeseed Oil

Directions

To alter mood for the better, add all ingredients to bathwater and stir to disperse. Inhale deeply while soaking for 20 minutes; avoid getting water in eyes.

Smooth Skin

Ingredients

4 drops Lavender Essential Oil

3 drops Bergamot Essential Oil

1 tsp Carrier Oil

Directions

For beautiful, smooth skin, combine all ingredients in a small container and mix well. Apply to the face or other affected area. Let sit for 5-10 minutes, then rinse with warm water.

Stimulating Bath

Ingredients

2 drops Bergamot Essential Oil

1 drop Patchouli Essential Oil

1 drop Rose Otto Essential Oil

1 Tbsp. Grapeseed Oil (optional)

Directions

To provide a burst of energy, add all ingredients to bathwater and stir to disperse. Inhale deeply while soaking for 20 minutes; avoid getting water in eyes.

Uplifting Massage Blend

Ingredients

20 mL Carrier Oil

3 drops Bergamot Essential Oil

3 drops Rosemary Essential Oil

3 drops Eucalyptus Essential Oil

3 drops Lime Essential Oil

3 drops Basil Essential Oil

5 drops Spearmint Essential Oil

Directions

For an uplifting massage, combine all oils in a small glass jar or container, cap with the lid, and shake until well blended. Use as normal.

Uplifting Massage Blend II

Ingredients

2 drops Bergamot Essential Oil

2 drops Geranium Essential Oil

2 drops Rosewood Essential Oil

6 tsps. Carrier Oil

Directions

Combine all ingredients in a small jar or bowl. When in need of a mood changer, massage the uplifting rub into the soles of the feet, or use for a full-body massage.

Uplifting Vaporizer Blend

Ingredients

4 drops Lemon Essential Oil

4 drops Bergamot Essential Oil

2 drops Tea Tree Essential Oil

Directions

To stabilize mood, diffuse the oils and breathe the vapors deeply.

Chapter 3:
Bergamot Essential Oil Studies

Many studies have been done on essential oils to discover and prove their therapeutic qualities. In the case of Bergamot studies, many of the properties attributed to the essential oil (noted in this book and elsewhere), are quite often validated through the scientific research of accredited universities, and published by accredited scientific journals. In this chapter we will discuss a small portion of these studies. It is important to note that research on essential oils is constant and evolving. Keep up with any recent research as it may turn up even further valuable uses of these miracle oils.

Study 1 – Anti-anxiety Properties

In this study, published by *Evidence-Based Complementary and Alternative Medicine*, the anti-anxiety effects of Bergamot essential oil were examined, with the following results: "The aim of this study was to determine if aromatherapy could reduce preoperative anxiety in ambulatory surgery patients...All those exposed to Bergamot essential oil aromatherapy showed a greater reduction in preoperative anxiety than those in the control groups. Aromatherapy may be a useful part of a holistic approach to reducing preoperative anxiety before ambulatory surgery."

In this study, 109 patients who were undergoing surgery were asked to participate in the study by filling out pre- and postoperative questionnaires – specifically the State Trait Anxiety Inventory (STAI), which asked the patients twenty questions, rating their level of anxiety, along with a recording of the patient's' vital signs. The patients were split into two groups, a control group and the experimental group, which received Bergamot aromatherapy pre-surgery.

The results showed that the heart rate, blood pressure, and STAI scores of the experimental group decreased significantly, indicating a reduction in preoperative anxiety. This suggests that aromatherapy, particularly that of Bergamot essential oil, may play a role in holistic nursing practices which aim to calm anxiety pre-surgery.

Reference:

Read the full text here:

Study 2 – Anticancer Properties

In this study, published by *PLOS One*, the anticancer effects of Bergamot essential oil were examined, with the following results: "Bergamot (Citrus bergamia, Risso et Poiteau) essential oil (BEO) is a well characterized, widely used plant extract. BEO exerts anxiolytic, analgesic and neuroprotective activities in rodents through mechanisms that are only partly known and need to be further investigated. To gain more insight into the biological effects of this essential oil, we tested the ability of BEO (0.005-0.03%) to modulate autophagic pathways in human SH-SY5Y neuroblastoma cells...The same features of stimulated autophagy elicited by BEO were reproduced by d-limonene, which rapidly increases LC3II and reduces p62 levels in a concentration-dependent manner. Linalyl acetate was ineffective in replicating BEO effects; however, it greatly enhanced LC3 lipidation triggered by d-limonene."

Neuroblastoma is cancer that occurs in infancy or childhood, most commonly in the extracranial, with around

650 cases occurring each year in America, nearly half in children under two years old. The tumor often occurs in an adrenal gland or in nerve tissue of the abdomen, pelvis, neck, or chest. Though the tumor may become malignant, it is most often low-risk in infants and can be treated through observation or surgery.

This study examined the effect of Bergamot essential oil on modulation of autophagic pathways in human SH-SY5Y neuroblastoma cells. Autophagy was induced by those cells treated with Bergamot. Autophagy is the basic mechanism, through the action of lysosomes, membrane-bound cell organelle which contain enzymes that induce cell degradation by breaking down dysfunctional cellular components. The Bergamot application also did not affect the phosphorylation of ULK1 (Ser757) and p70S6K (Thr389), two protein enzymes. The study indicates that Bergamot essential oil may supplement the body's defenses against neuroblastoma cells. It also indicates that d-limonene and linalyl acetate, in combination, were the components of the oil most likely responsible for its positive effects.

Reference:
http://www.ncbi.nlm.nih.gov/pubmed/25419658]

http://www.ncbi.nlm.nih.gov/pmc/articles/PMC4242674/pdf/pone.0113682.pdf]

Study 3 – Antibacterial Properties

In this study, available on PubMed, the antibacterial effects of Bergamot essential oil on MRSA were examined, with the following results: "Antibiotic-resistant organisms such as meticillin-resistant Staphylococcus aureus (MRSA) and vancomycin-resistant Enterococcus sp. (VRE) are an ongoing problem in hospitals. Essential oil vapors (EOs) have been shown to reduce environmental bacterial contamination...Citrus vapor has potential for application in the clinical environment, for instance as a secondary disinfectant to reduce surface contamination by VRE and MRSA."

This study aimed to assess the efficacy of a blend of vaporized essential oils – including orange and Bergamot – on eliminating Staphylococcus aureus and Enterococcus sp., from stainless steel surfaces, like those in hospitals, where MRSA can spread if untreated.

Staphylococcus aureus is a gram-positive bacterium. Although Staphylococcus aureus is part of the normal human skin flora and the respiratory tract, it is not typically pathogenic when it becomes so. Staphylococcus aureus produces respiratory issues like sinusitis, skin infections, and even food poisoning. Those with compromised immune systems are particularly vulnerable to the bacteria and can potentially develop an infection. Enterococcus species are also gram positive bacterium which can result in clinical infections that include bacteremia, diverticulitis, meningitis, bacterial endocarditis, and urinary tract infections. These bacteria are highly resistant and prove an endemic problem in some hospitals.

The study examined the citrus vapor's effect on the bacteria biofilms and found that, after 24 hours of exposure, the vapor reduced MRSA and VRE on stainless steel surfaces by 1.5-3log (10). These results suggest that citrus vapor can be applied as a secondary disinfectant in clinical environments to decrease contamination by these bacteria.

Reference
http://www.ncbi.nlm.nih.gov/pubmed/22153952]

Study 4 – Neuropathic Hypersensitivity

In this study available on PubMed, the effects of Bergamot essential oil on neuropathic hypersensitivity were examined, with the following results: "Bergamot essential oil (BEO) is one of the most common essential oil containing linalool and linalyl acetate as major volatile components. This study investigated the effect of intraplantar (i.pl.) Bergamot essential oil (BEO) or linalool on neuropathic hypersensitivity induced by partial sciatic nerve ligation (PSNL) in mice...In western blotting analysis, i.pl. injection of BEO or linalool resulted in a significant blockade of spinal ERK activation induced by PSNL. These results suggest that i.pl. injection of BEO or linalool may reduce

PSNL-induced mechanical allodynia followed by decreasing spinal ERK activation."

Resulting from diseases that impact the somatosensory system, neuropathic pain affects significant numbers of the global population and may be associated with pain caused by normally non-painful stimuli. Qualities of neuropathic hypersensitivity include "pins and needles" sensations, itching, numbness, and cold or burning sensations. Neuropathic pain may be chronic or episodic, like electric shocks, and is often caused by disorders of the central nervous system (brain or spinal cord).

This study examined the effects of Bergamot essential oil on neuropathic hypersensitivity, particularly that of ERK activation in the spine, which results in an inflammatory factors and noxious pain. The results of the study indicate that the injection of Bergamot essential oil blocked the ERK activation, thereby alleviating neuropathic hypersensitivity when it comes to spinal pain. The study also indicates that linalool, one of Bergamot's chemical components, is active in reducing spinal ERK activation.

Reference
http://www.ncbi.nlm.nih.gov/pubmed/23159543]

Study 5 – Cardiovascular Disease

In this study, available on PubMed, the effect of Bergamot essential oil on vascular smooth muscles were examined, with the following results: "In this study, we compared the effect of the essential oil of Citrus bergamia Risso [Bergamot, Bergamot essential oil (BEO)] on the intracellular Ca levels in vascular endothelial (EA) and mouse vascular smooth muscle (MOVAS) cells, using the fura-2 fluorescence technique...The present results suggest that BEO and LA differentially modulate intracellular Ca levels in vascular endothelial and smooth muscle cells. In addition, blockade of Ca influx by BEO and LA in EA cells may explain the protective effects of BEO on endothelial dysfunction associated with cardiovascular disease."

Vascular smooth muscle composes most of the blood vessel wall, and contracts to lower blood pressure by changing the volume of the wall's blood vessels. Vascular smooth muscle helps to redistribute the body's blood to regions where it is most needed, such as regions where oxygen consumption has temporarily increased. High blood pressure contributes to hypertension and cardiovascular disease, which is the leading cause of death, worldwide.

This results of the study indicate that Bergamot essential oil, and particularly, its major component linalyl acetate, helped block Ca influx in endothelial cells, which may support the body's natural defenses against the endothelial dysfunction linked to cardiovascular disease.

Reference & Photo Credit:
http://www.ncbi.nlm.nih.gov/pubmed/23288200]

Study 6 – Stress

A second study published by *Evidence-Based Complementary and Alternative Medicine* examined the effects of Bergamot essential oil on stress, with the following results: "Workplace stress-related illness is a serious issue, and consequently many stress reduction methods have been investigated. Aromatherapy is especially for populations that work under high stress. Elementary school teachers are a high-stress working population in Taiwan. In this study, fifty-four elementary school teachers were recruited to evaluate aromatherapy performance on stress reduction...All parameters were significantly different for most subgroups, except for the substitute teachers and the light-anxiety group. Parasympathetic nervous system activation was measured after aromatherapy in this study."

Similar to the first study, physiological records, including heart rate and blood pressure, were kept for each session of aromatherapy, documenting the participants' vital signs. The results showed that the heart rate and blood pressure of those undergoing aromatherapy decreased significantly, indicating a reduction in stress or anxiety. This suggests that aromatherapy, particularly that of Bergamot essential oil, may support a more balanced state in autonomic nervous activity

Reference
http://www.ncbi.nlm.nih.gov/pubmed/21584196]

http://www.ncbi.nlm.nih.gov/pmc/articles/PMC3092730/
pdf/ECAM2011-946537.pdf]

Chapter 4:
The Ins & Outs of Essential Oils

Where do essential oils come from?

Plants and plant species naturally produce essential oils for various reasons, one being to draw pollinator insects to them, another being to repel invading organisms (bacteria, animals). A number of chemical compounds compose each plant's essential oil, and the combination of these compounds are specific to each oil, which then instills in the oil its own unique properties. Essential oils can be harnessed from all sorts of plant components, including flowers, leaves, bark, fruit, roots, and resin. For instance, cinnamon oil is harnessed from bark, lemon oil from the peel, and lavender oil from flowers. Certain plants can produce a few chemical variants of the same essential oil, which are acquired from different parts of the plant. Some of these parts produce a large amount of oil, while others produce just a smidgen. The oil's quality and potency depends upon a number of factors, including the subspecies of the plant, its soil conditions, the time of year, and even the time of day you harvest it.

How are essential oils extracted?

Essential oils can be extracted from plants through various methods, including pressing, distillation, solvent, and maceration. Let's take a brief look at each:

Pressing Method

Commonly used with citrus fruit, the pressing method extracts the oil through a technique which involves pushing the fruit peels through a press. Oily fruits and plants are best suited for this technique. Orange oil, for example, is extracted from orange skins through the pressing method.

Distillation Method

This technique harkens back to the days of moonshiners, as the same sort of method used to create strong liquor can be used to extract essential oils. Using a still, boiled water, and plant materials, will create steam which is then cooled by coils and condensed into a combination of water and oil. This combination does not mix, so the oil can then be extracted from it.

Solvent Method

Through a multi-step process, certain plant and flower oils can be extracted using alcohol and other solvents, which extract the essential oils from the plant materials.

Maceration Method

When a "carrier," fixed oil, or lard is mixed with the plant material and set out in the sun over a period of time, the carrier oil is infused with the plant's essence. Heat sources, other than the sun, are often used to speed the process. Throughout the process more plant material is added to produce a more potent oil.

How do you use essential oils?

Although some studies about the effectiveness of essential oils are conducted by small companies, or even individuals, a number of them are conducted by the food and cosmetic industries. In general, the pharmaceutical industry shows next to no interest in herbal medicine, primarily because there are few options to patent such products. As such, the product's lack of profitability results in a lack of research funding. Regardless, the historical uses of essential oils tell us what we need to know; these oils have been effectively administered for centuries. The therapeutic qualifications of essential oils can be plotted in the survival of the human race across cultures and generations.

Another reason that studies on essential oils have not resulted in much conclusive evidence as to their overall effectiveness is because definitive results are sometimes difficult to prove, as the quality of each batch of oil can vary for a number of reasons. One is that essential oils are impossible to standardize. As mentioned above, even the slightest variance in soil conditions, and the time of harvesting – as well as innumerable other factors – will produce a different product quality and potency. In addition, essential oils are often obtained from various species of the same plant; Eucalyptus radiata and Eucalyptus globulus can both be used in the making of therapeutic-grade eucalyptus oil, as a result, they may have slightly different properties and degrees of strength or effectiveness.

Just as there are a number of methods by which to extract essential oils, there are a number of methods to administer them therapeutically. The variety of chemical compounds in each essential oil means that their benefits and applications also vary across the board. Below are a few of these methods.

Topical Administration

Direct application of many essential oils works like a sponge, as skin absorbs chemicals and other things (like sunlight, for instance). Topical application is best for clearing up an ailment on the skin's surface, or in the underlying muscle tissue. When applying topically, massage the oil into the skin, or simply dab on the skin for therapeutic results. Combine the essential oil with a carrier oil for topical use in order to dilute its potency. This is safer as the oil is concentrated. Support the body's defenses against rash or muscle pain in this manner, but always test the patient for allergies before applying. Adverse effects are produced by natural chemicals as much as synthetic ones; poison ivy, for example.

To test for allergens, place a drop or two on the patient's inner forearm. If a rash develops within 12 to 24 hours, then the patient is allergic. In addition, phototoxicity – sun exposure resulting in an exacerbated burn – may be an issue when citrus oils are applied topically. One must proceed with caution when applying essential oils using this method.

Inhalation Therapy

Commonly known as "aromatherapy," this essential oil application is effective for inner ailments, like sore throat, or cold. In a steaming bowl of distilled, or sterilized water, add a few drops of essential oil, then with a towel over your head, bend over the bowl and inhale. The towel captures the vapors, making the technique even more effective. Essential oils can also be placed in a diffuser, or potpourri throughout a room, to produce somewhat diluted medicinal effects.

Ingestion

When using this method, proceed with caution. Direct ingestion of essential oils must be monitored and applied in small doses that are diluted in a tablespoon or more of any carrier oil – olive oil, for example. If you are unsure of dosage amounts, make a tea with the relevant herb instead.

Although the effects of this diluted use may be weaker, this application is a better alternative than an overdose of essential oils.

What are the general benefits of using essential oils?

Replacement for Prescription Drugs

One practical benefit of using essential oils is their substitutive nature; they can replace Rx drugs, which is the ultimate reason to learn about their administration, and begin stockpiling an essential oil supply. One of the potential threats of economic/social collapse is the lack of resources, and primarily the inability to procure prescription drugs. As such, finding suitable alternatives should be a priority when prepping for the worst.

Their portability is also a major bonus when it comes to survival prepping. The fact that these ultra-concentrated oils take up little-to-no space makes toting them all the simpler should the need arise. Because essential oils are highly concentrated, the application used in most methods of administration requires only a drop or two of oil, which means that tiny bottle will last a long time.

Cheap, but Effective Alternative

Though money may be the last thing on your mind when it comes to prepping for a survival situation (money may even be obsolete in the event of social collapse), it is worth noting that the expense of essential oils pales in comparison to prescription drugs. Essential oils are an inexpensive, yet equally effective alternative to prescription medicine.

No Expiration Date

Another benefit of essential oils is that they do not expire, nor do they have "proper storage" requirements. A number of medicines, and medicinal products, must be replaced every few years; this sets essential oils ahead of the pack when it comes to shelf life.

Versatility

Essential oils also offer great versatility. Aside from providing health benefits, essential oils can be repurposed for household and hygienic applications. For instance, if looking for something that might serve dental hygiene needs in a time of crisis, then thieves oil is a go-to essential oil. To maintain the skin's health, frankincense and lavender will do the trick; the latter also serves as sunscreen, preventing sun damage as well.

When it comes to the house or shelter, use essential oils to deodorize, which will come in handy in a disaster scenario, especially if things start to smell due to lack of proper utilities and maintenance. For example, after the 2011 tsunami and the subsequent nuclear reactor meltdown in Japan, a nurse named Risa Nakahira used essential oils to deodorize and sanitize putrid public bathrooms in overpopulated evacuation facilities. As relief workers searched for survivors, often wading through debris and decay, Nakahira also deodorized their boots and masks using essential oils. The possibilities of these natural oils are endless.

They are also versatile when it comes to the range of patients they are capable of supporting. The health of everyone, from a great grandfather to an infant baby, can be fortified with the aid of essential oils in the appropriate dosage. They even come in handy when treating livestock or pets. From teething infants to dementia in the elderly, from teenagers with acne to dogs with urinary tract infections, essential oils can serve any patient with nearly any ailment.

Conclusion

Now that you know all about what Bergamot essential oil can do for you – where it originates, how it is extracted, the benefits and properties, and the different methods of administration – use it confidently to support the body's defenses against health issues and start to assemble a kit of essential oils for survival. Essential oils can be purchased online or at your local holistic treatment store.

The various benefits of essential oils and their properties are countless. To build a kit, first focus on acquiring the essential oils which may bear more relevance to personal health issues, or the potential health threats, within the environment. In the event of a viral outbreak, for instance, Bergamot essential oil will be one of the more crucial oils – along with oregano, lemon, frankincense, and cinnamon (eBooks also available for purchase) – due to their antiviral and immuno-supportive properties.

Used as a supplement or as the go-to for skin conditions, infections, or immune-boosting agents, the application of Bergamot essential oil in medicine has survived for centuries and will survive centuries more. When it comes down to it, we do not need to rely on pharmaceuticals; essential oils, herbs, and plenty of other natural ingredients can be used to help support the body's natural defenses against any number of health issues; ailment or injury.

Essential oils are essential to your survival in the case

of viral outbreak, social collapse, or natural disaster because, when the SHTF, access to pharmaceuticals will likely be limited, or obsolete altogether. Alternatives to our modern-day standard will equate survival when no other option exists

DISCLAIMER AND/OR LEGAL NOTICES: Every effort has been made to accurately represent this book and it's potential. Results vary with every individual, and your results may or may not be different from those depicted. No promises, guarantees or warranties, whether stated or implied, have been made that you will produce any specific result from this book. Your efforts are individual and unique, and may vary from those shown. Your success depends on your efforts, background and motivation.

The material in this publication is provided for educational and informational purposes only and is not intended as medical advice. The information contained in this book should not be used to diagnose or treat any illness, metabolic disorder, disease or health problem. Always consult your physician or healthcare provider before beginning any nutrition or exercise program. Use of the programs, advice, and information contained in this book is at the sole choice and risk of the reader.